SHORT-TERM MONITORING OF FORMALDEHYDE: COMPARISON OF TWO DIRECT-READING INSTRUMENTS TO A LABORATORY-BASED METHOD

Deborah V.L. Myers, Ph.D., E.I.
Chad H. Dowell, M.S., C.I.H.
and
Michael G. Gressel, Ph.D., C.S.P.
NIOSH

W. Dana Flanders, M.D., D.Sc.
National Center for Environmental Health

I0493914

REPORT DATE:

June 2009

REPORT NO.:

EPHB 331-05b

MANUSCRIPT PREPARED BY:

Bernice Clark

U.S. Department of Health and Human Services
Public Health Service
Centers for Disease Control and Prevention
National Institute for Occupational safety and Health
Division of Applied Research and Technology
4676 Columbia Parkway, MS-R5
Cincinnati, Ohio 45226

SITE SURVEYED: Selfield Industrial Park
                                        Federal Emergency Management Agency
                                        Selma, Alabama

SURVEY DATE: July 28–31, 2008

SURVEY CONDUCTED BY: Deborah V.L. Myers, Ph.D, E.I.
                                        NIOSH
                                        Cincinnati, OH

                                        Michael G. Gressel, Ph.D., C.S.P.
                                        NIOSH
                                        Cincinnati, OH

                                        Gary P. Noonan, M.P.A.
                                        National Center for Environmental Health/
                                        Division of Environmental Hazards and
                                        Health Effects
                                        Atlanta, GA

                                        Ronald Dobos, C.I.H., C.S.P.
                                        Bureau Veritas North America, Inc.
                                        Kennesaw, GA

                                        William Dendy, REM
                                        Bureau Veritas North America, Inc.
                                        Kennesaw, GA

SITE REPRESENTATIVES
CONTACTED: Ronald Parten, Site Manager
                                        Selma, AL

                                        Randy Brown
                                        Selma, AL

DISCLAIMER

Mention of company names or products does not constitute endorsement by the Centers for Disease Control and Prevention.

The findings and conclusions in this report are those of the authors and do not necessarily represent the views of the National Institute for Occupational Safety and Health and the National Center for Environmental Health.

ACKNOWLEDGEMENTS

The authors gratefully acknowledge the significant collaboration of CDC and Bureau Veritas North America for this work. Field guidance, data collection, and data analysis were provided by Gary Noonan, Liane Hostler, Rick Aspray, Ronald Dobos, William Dendy, Paul Epstein, Sam Tucker, Dan Farwick, Kevin H. Dunn, Dave Marlow, Brenda Jones, Debbie Fite, Teresa Lewis, Donald Booher, and Karl Feldmann. Field site assistance was provided by Ronald Parten, Randy Brown, and other site personnel. Editorial assistance was provided by Ellen Galloway.

ABSTRACT

Formaldehyde is used in the production of many household and building products and its health hazards are well recognized. Airborne formaldehyde concentrations can be measured using several different techniques, including laboratory-based methods and direct-reading instruments. For this study, two commercially available direct-reading instruments, an RKI Instruments Model FP-30 and a PPM Technology Formaldemeter[™] htV, were compared with NIOSH Method 2016 in different test environments to determine if these direct-reading instruments can accurately measure formaldehyde. The RKI Instruments Model FP-30 instrument uses photoelectric photometry technology to measure formaldehyde, while the PPM Technology Formaldemeter[™] htV instrument uses electrochemical sensing technology. NIOSH Method 2016 is an integrated sampling method that collects formaldehyde on silica gel coated with 2,4-dinitrophenylhydrazine; the derivitized product (2,4-dinitrophenylhydrazone) is analyzed using high performance liquid chromatography with UV detection. Forty-seven 1-hour integrated air samples were collected and analyzed for formaldehyde using NIOSH Method 2016. Measurements were made simultaneously with both direct-reading instruments and with the NIOSH Method. The methods yielded the following mean concentrations for the 47 samples: NIOSH Method 2016, 0.37 ppm; RKI Instruments Model FP-30, 0.29 ppm; and PPM Technology Formaldemeter[™] htV, 0.340 ppm. Pearson correlation showed that the NIOSH Method and the PPM Technology Formaldemeter[™] htV ($R^2 = 0.902$) were more associated than the NIOSH Method and the RKI Instruments Model FP-30 ($R^2 = 0.780$). Comparison of 1-hour integrated samples from the three methods showed that on average the RKI Instruments Model FP-30 instrument ($p<0.001$) differed significantly from the NIOSH Method 2016, whereas the PPM Technology Formaldemeter[™] htV ($p=0.15$) was not significantly different from the NIOSH

Method. Sensitivity and specificity tests demonstrated that 1-hour integrated samples with the PPM Technology Formaldemeter™ *htV* was more accurate at measuring formaldehyde concentrations greater than 0.2 ppm, while the RKI Instruments Model FP-30 was better at measuring concentrations less than 0.2 ppm. Although the direct-reading instruments differed from NIOSH Method 2016, scatter plots and correlation tests showed that the 1-hour integrated sample collected with the direct-reading instruments correlated with those from the laboratory-based method.

Table of Contents

Figures

Tables

INTRODUCTION

Formaldehyde (HCOH) is a colorless, pungent-smelling gas at room temperature [Pickrell et al. 1983]. It is used in the manufacturing of many products, such as plywood, paper, resins, fertilizers, cosmetics, and medications, and in household products as a preservative [ATSDR 1999; Kelly et al. 1999; Khoder et al. 2000]. Formaldehyde is commonly released into the air by burning wood or natural gas, from cigarettes or automobiles exhaust, or by off-gassing from certain materials [U.S. Consumer Product Safety Commission 1997; Khoder et al. 2000]. Formaldehyde is a suspect human carcinogen and a respiratory and skin sensitizer [Khoder et al. 2000]. Formaldehyde concentrations in the environment above the National Institute for Occupational Safety and Health (NIOSH) recommended exposure limit (REL) of 0.016 parts per million (ppm), can cause eye, skin, and respiratory tract irritation [NIOSH 2005]. Formaldehyde use in various building products such as urea formaldehyde foam insulation and wood products has led to research on its off-gassing rate in mobile homes and other consumer products [Pickrell et al. 1983].

Airborne formaldehyde can be measured using different techniques, such as laboratory-based methods and direct-reading instruments. Direct-reading instruments provide results real-time or within a few minutes; laboratory-based methods, which necessitate sample analysis, can typically take up to 2 weeks for results. However, comparisons of the reliability and accuracy of direct-reading methods to a fully evaluated air sampling method for airborne formaldehyde concentrations are limited. The objective of this study was to compare two direct-reading formaldehyde instruments in a field application to determine if the direct-reading instruments can provide accurate measurements. The study compared the RKI Instruments Model FP-30 and the

PPM Technology Formaldemeter™ *htV* with fully evaluated NIOSH Method 2016 [NIOSH 2003]. The null hypothesis for the study was that the mean formaldehyde concentration for each direct-reading instrument would be equal to the mean concentration measured by NIOSH Method 2016.

METHODS

This field survey provided an opportunity to compare two commercially available direct-reading instruments to NIOSH Method 2016 for measuring formaldehyde in air. The direct-reading instruments used in the comparison study were the RKI Instruments Model FP-30 and the PPM Technology Formaldemeter™ *htV*. A brief search was conducted to find formaldehyde direct-reading instruments. Based on cost and availability, the RKI Instruments Model FP-30 and the PPM Technology Formaldemeter™ *htV* were chosen for this study. Details of the three methods are presented in Table 1 [Peluffo 2009; Roberts 2009]. For tabulated data, the analytical methods are referred to as NIOSH (NIOSH Method 2016), RKI (RKI Instruments Model FP-30), PPM (PPM Technology Formaldemeter™ *htV*), HPLC (high performance liquid chromatography), UV (Ultraviolet), R^2 (coefficient of determination), SD (standard deviation), SE (standard error), and N (number of observations).

Table 1. Formaldehyde Method Characteristics

	NIOSH	RKI	PPM
Analytical Technique	HPLC, UV detection	Photoelectric photometry	Electrochemical
Range	0.23 to 37 μg/sample	0 to 1.00 ppm	0 to 10.00 ppm
Accuracy	± 19%	± 10%	± 25%
Interferants	Ozone, ketones, other aldehydes	None reported	Phenol, resorcinol, alcohols, aldehydes, humidity >60%
Flow Rate	0.030 to 1.5 L/min	0.35 L/min	0.353 L/min
Sample Period	60 min	15 min	60 sec[*]

[*]60 seconds in high accuracy mode and 8 seconds in low accuracy mode. For this study, the PPM was in high accuracy mode.

Description of the Direct-Reading Instruments and Laboratory-Based Method

Direct-Reading Instruments

The RKI Instruments Model FP-30 uses photoelectric photometry with colorimetric detection tabs to measure formaldehyde in air (RKI Instruments Inc., Hayward, California) (Figure A-1 in Appendix). The RKI Instruments Model FP-30 draws in air with an internal pump and uses a microprocessor to control sample flow rate. The instrument uses detection tabs to sample airborne formaldehyde. Depending on the desired detection range, a particular tab number is used during sampling. For this study, number 009 detection tabs were used to measure formaldehyde concentrations ranging from 0 to 1.00 ppm in a 15-minute sampling time. The instruction manual states the RKI Instruments Model FP-30 is capable of measuring formaldehyde concentrations ranging from 0 to 1.00 ppm with a resolution of 0.01 ppm. According to the manufacturer, measurements are accurate to ± 10% when air temperature is between 14°F and 104°F and the relative humidity is below 90%.

The PPM Technology Formaldemeter[™] *htV* uses electrochemical sensing technology to measure airborne formaldehyde concentrations (PPM Technology Ltd., Caernarfon, Gwynedd, Wales,

United Kingdom) (Figure A-2 in Appendix). The Formaldemeter™ *htV* collects single air samples upon initiation by the user, uses a sampling frequency of 1 to 3 minutes, and analyzes the samples within 60 seconds. The operation manual states the Formaldemeter™ *htV* is capable of measuring formaldehyde concentrations ranging from 0 to 10.00 ppm with resolution of 0.001 ppm. Phenol is a positive interference for the Formaldemeter™ *htV* [PPM Technology Ltd 2005]. To prevent potential sensor interference by phenol, samples were collected with an inline phenol filter according to the manufacturer's instructions. The filters can remove phenols from the air sample without affecting the reading. Alcohols and aldehydes can also cause interference to the monitor. As noted by the manufacturer [PPM Technology Ltd 2005], the PPM Technology Formaldemeter™ *htV* is sensitive to high temperatures and humidity. Relative humidity above 60% could cause a background reading on the instrument. The PPM Technology Formaldemeter™ *htV* is specially designed to compensate for relative humidity above 60% using data analysis functions. Also, the instrument is temperature compensated to operate accurately in the range of 50°F–86°F. Generally formaldehyde concentrations increase with increasing temperatures in the environment being evaluated [Roberts 2009]. Between the temperatures 50-86°F, all results fall within ± 25% of the true value at the 95% confidence level for the instrument, above 86°F the results are still linear (i.e., as temperature increases, the instrument gives a higher reading) and can be used as a good guideline but the results do deviate from ideal [Roberts 2009].

Laboratory-Based Method

NIOSH Method 2016 was used as the reference method for comparison of the two direct-reading instruments. This method is fully evaluated which included testing to quantify storage stability, collection efficiency, and breakthrough volumes [NIOSH 1995]. In order to be fully evaluated, a

NIOSH method must meet a ± 25% accuracy criterion at a 95% confidence level. NIOSH

Method 2016 requires that air samples be collected using a cartridge containing silica gel coated

with 2,4-dinitrophenylhydrazine (2,4-DNPH). For this study, samples were collected on Supelco

S10 LpDNPH cartridges [model #S10L, lot #SP9984]. Because ozone can consume the 2,4-

DNPH reagent and degrade the formaldehyde derivative [NIOSH 2003], a Supelco LpDNPH

ozone scrubber was used with each air sample cartridge. The Supelco LpDNPH ozone scrubber

was connected upstream of the S10L cartridge, which was connected via plastic tubing to the

inlet port of an SKC AirCheck® 2000 sampling pump (SKC Limited, Harrisburg, Pennsylvania)

(pump shown in Figure A-3 in Appendix). All SKC AirCheck® 2000 pumps were calibrated

with a Bios DryCal® DC-Lite (BIOS, Butler, New Jersey) to a flow rate of 0.5 liters per minute

(L/min). Multiple samples were collected with the same pumps throughout the day. Each

collected sample and field blank were immediately capped and placed in individual metallized

packaging to protect the media from air, moisture, and light. The ozone scrubbers were

discarded after each sample. At the end of each sampling day, the samples and field blanks were

shipped on ice (0°C), according to the method, to the contracting laboratory for analysis. All

samples were analyzed by Bureau Veritas North America, Novi, Michigan. Pre- and post-

sampling pump flow checks were performed at the beginning and end of the sampling day.

NIOSH Method 2016 laboratory sample results were reported in micrograms (μg) per sample

and parts per billion (ppb). Based on the W-test of log-transformed concentration data, the data

distribution was determined to be lognormal (p=0.961). Therefore, samples with concentrations

below the minimum detectable concentration (MDC) were noted and replaced with the MDC

divided by the square root of 2 [Hornung and Reed 1990]. The MDC is defined as the limit of detection (LOD) divided by the sample volume. The MDC was 2.0 ppb with a 28 L average sample volume collected over one hour.

For each test location, ambient temperature and relative humidity were measured using a calibrated VelociCalc Plus monitor (Model 8386A, TSI Incorporated, Shoreview, Minnesota). This instrument provides real-time temperature and relative humidity measurements.

Test Environment

Results of the Sexton et al. [1989] study suggested manufactured homes and similar structures, such as temporary housing units (THU) that were purchased by the Federal Emergency Management Agency (FEMA) for use as temporary housing during national emergency events, were an appropriate environment for conducting a study comparing two direct-reading instruments for formaldehyde. For convenience and access to different types of THUs, this study was conducted at the FEMA storage site at Selfield Industrial Park in Selma, Alabama where a variety of manufactured homes, park homes, and travel trailers were stored. The three sampling methods—the two direct-reading instruments and the NIOSH analytical method—were used in each type of THU and represent a sample set. The different THUs were tested in either ventilated (windows or doors opened) or unventilated (windows or doors closed) configurations to provide a wide range of formaldehyde concentrations. The ventilation state was not used as a variable in data analysis. Providing ventilation decreases formaldehyde concentrations, while closed units would most likely result in higher concentrations [U.S. Consumer Product Safety Commission 1997]. A convenience sample of THUs was used for this study. Sampling personnel remained in the THUs for the duration of each sample and wore suitable respiratory protection.

Test Procedure

All three formaldehyde sampling methods (i.e., sample set) were simultaneously started within one minute of entering each THU. Ambient temperature and relative humidity measurements were recorded at the same time with the VelociCalc Plus monitor. All samples were collected side-by-side in the center of each unit, near or in the kitchen. A 1-hour area air sample for formaldehyde was collected in each of the THUs in accordance with NIOSH Method 2016 for a nominal 30 L sample volume. The sampling period for all methods was 1-hour. Because of the differences in the operation of the instruments, the NIOSH Method 2016, the RKI Instruments Model FP-30, and the PPM Technology Formaldemeter™ *htV* collected a different number of samples during the sampling period. For the direct-reading instruments, these samples were averaged over the 1-hour sampling period for comparison among the three methods. Three samples for formaldehyde were collected using the RKI Instruments Model FP-30. Samples were started every 18 minutes throughout the 1-hour sampling period. The means for the three RKI Instruments Model FP-30 samples were used in the analysis. The detection tabs were discarded after each use. Five samples were collected every 12 minutes using the PPM Technology Formaldemeter™ *htV* and the means for the five samples were used in the analysis. The phenol filter was replaced and discarded every fifth sample (as specified in the manufacturer's instructions).

A standardized sample collection data sheet was used to document relevant sampling data and notes (Figures A-4 and A-5 in the Appendix). Information included sample start and stop times, location of sample collection, pump/instrument information, formaldehyde concentrations (in ppm), and ambient temperature and relative humidity.

Data Analysis

Initially, the data were analyzed using descriptive statistics including means, medians, standard deviations, and minimum and maximum values. Paired t-tests were used to compare the average differences among the methods. The association between NIOSH Method 2016 and the two direct-reading instruments was assessed by bivariate scatter plots, Bland-Altman plots, correlation analyses, and linear regression. The Spearman and Pearson correlation coefficients were used as measures of the strength of the association between the formaldehyde values obtained from the different methods. The sensitivity and specificity of the two direct-reading instruments were assessed to detect a level above 0.2 ppm by using NIOSH Method 2016 as the reference concentration method. For the sensitivity and specificity tests, 0.2 ppm was chosen as the arbitrary cutoff level. The predictive ability of the direct-reading instruments was further assessed by using each, separately, to predict a level above 0.2 ppm according to NIOSH Method 2016 and calculating the area under the curve. Regression diagnostics included evaluation of squared terms, use of condition indices to assess potential collinearity, and residual plots. In sensitivity analyses, results analyzed using a log-transform obtained qualitatively similar results as the regression diagnostics. All analyses were done in Microsoft Excel software (2003,

15

Microsoft Corporation, Redmond, Washington) and SAS (9.1, SAS Institute Inc., Cary, North

Carolina).

RESULTS

A total of 72 sample sets were collected using each of the three sampling methods (RKI

Instruments Model FP-30, PPM Technology Formaldemeter™ *htV*, and NIOSH Method 2016).

However, only 47 sample sets were included in the analysis because some of the sampling

pumps used for the NIOSH Method 2016 had pre- and post-sampling flow rate differences

greater than 10%. To address this flow rate problem, only the first and last samples of a

sequence of samples from the same pump with greater than 10% difference in pre- and post-

sampling flow rates were included in the analysis. The concentration for the first sample was

calculated using the pre-sampling flow rate, while the concentration for the last sample was

calculated using the post-sampling flow rate. All other samples with flow rate differences of

10% or less were included in the analysis using the mean of the pre- and post-sampling flow

rates. However, the overall research findings did not change when the mean flow rate value was

applied to the original 72 sample sets (Table A-1 in the Appendix). Results for the direct-

reading instruments were integrated and reported as an average of the three measurements for the

RKI Instruments Model FP-30 and five measurements for the PPM Technology Formaldemeter™

htV.

Direct-Reading Instruments versus NIOSH Method 2016

Table 2 presents descriptive statistics for each sampling method. RKI Instruments Model FP-30

data ranged from 0.01 to 1.00 ppm, the upper limit for the monitor, with a mean of 0.29 ppm.

PPM Technology Formaldemeter™ *htV* data ranged from 0.032 to 1.220 ppm with an average value of 0.341 ppm. NIOSH Method 2016 data ranged from 0.026 to 1.5 ppm with an average of 0.37 ppm. The RKI Instruments Model FP-30 and NIOSH Method 2016 had a mean difference of 0.09 ppm (p=0.0007), while the NIOSH Method 2016 and PPM Technology Formaldemeter™ *htV* had a mean difference of 0.030 ppm (p=0.15). Five sample results from the RKI Instruments Model FP-30 were recorded as 1.00 ppm, the maximum for the monitor. If these five samples results from the RKI Instruments Model FP-30 and the associated data points from the NIOSH Method 2016 and PPM Technology Formaldemeter™ *htV* are excluded from the analyzed data set, then the mean values for the 42 observations for the NIOSH Method 2016, RKI Instruments Model FP-30, and PPM Technology Formaldemeter™ *htV* methods are 0.29, 0.20, and 0.281 ppm, respectively (Table A-2 in Appendix).

Table 2. Summary Statistics for NIOSH, RKI, and PPM Sampling Methods

Method Paired Triplets	N	Mean (SD) (ppm)	Mean Difference vs NIOSH (SD) (ppm)	Median (ppm)	Min/Max (ppm)	Max-Min Difference (ppm)	Mean[*] Squared Error
NIOSH	47	0.37 (0.35)	—	0.22	0.026 1.5	1.5	—
RKI	47	0.29 (0.32)	0.09 (0.16)	0.07	0.01 1.00	0.99	0.03
PPM	47	0.341 (0.240)	0.030 (0.140)	0.246	0.032 1.220	1.188	0.019

[*] NIOSH as the reference value for this analysis

The Spearman correlation was used to test the nonparametric correlation between the direct-reading instruments and NIOSH Method 2016, while the Pearson correlation coefficient was used to measure the linear relationship between the methods. Table 3 shows the correlation coefficients for the different methods. The Pearson correlation coefficient for the RKI

Instruments Model FP-30 and NIOSH Method 2016 was 0.780, and 0.902 for the PPM

Technology Formaldemeter™ *htV* and NIOSH Method 2016. The Spearman correlation

coefficient for the RKI Instruments Model FP-30 and NIOSH Method 2016 was 0.883, and

0.949 for the PPM Technology Formaldemeter™ *htV* and NIOSH Method 2016. Figure 1

presents a scatter plot and the regression line for the RKI instrument versus NIOSH Method

2016. Figure 2 presents a scatter plot and regression line for the PPM instrument versus NIOSH

Method 2016. Figure 3 shows a scatter plot and regression line for the two direct-reading

instruments.

Table 3. Correlation Coefficients for NIOSH, RKI, and PPM Sampling Methods

Method	NIOSH Pearson/Spearman	RKI Pearson/Spearman	PPM Pearson/Spearman
NIOSH	1 / 1	0.780 / 0.883	0.902 / 0.949
RKI	0.780 / 0.883	1 / 1	0.699 / 0.836
PPM	0.902 / 0.949	0.699 / 0.836	1 / 1

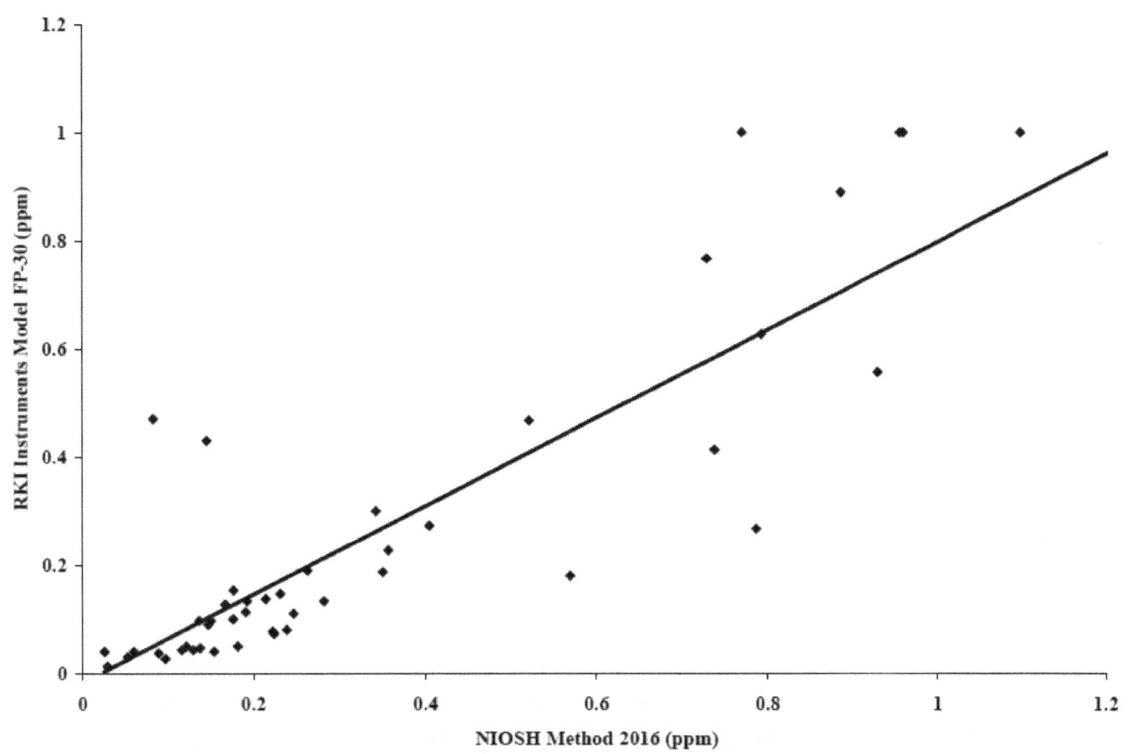

Figure 1. Scatter Plot of RKI Instruments Model FP-30 versus NIOSH Method 2016

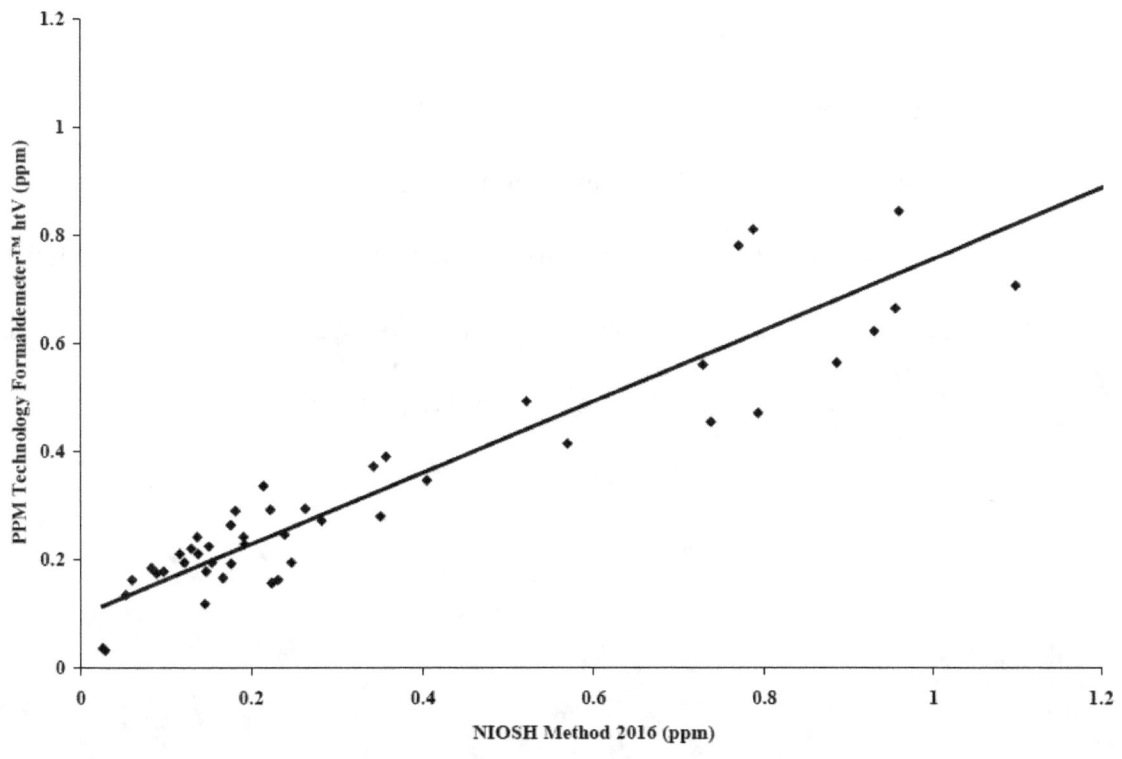

Figure 2. Scatter Plot of PPM Technology Formaldemeter[TM] ***htV* versus NIOSH Method 2016**

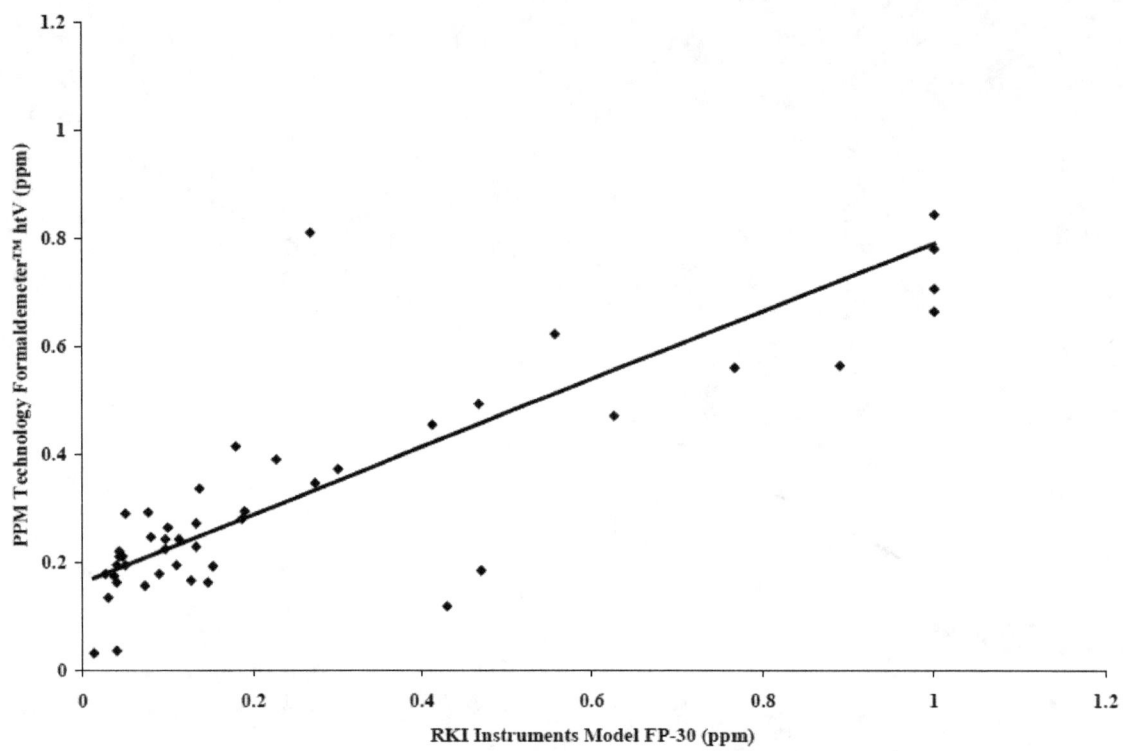

Figure 3. Scatter Plot of PPM Technology Formaldemeter™ *htV* versus RKI Instruments Model FP-30

Table 4 displays the multiple linear regression summary of the three methods with additional parameters, temperature and relative humidity. Temperature and relative humidity were added to the model to determine if the parameters influenced the relationship between the NIOSH Method and each of the two direct-reading instruments. Bland-Altman plots were done with all methods (Figures A-6 through A-8 in the Appendix) to measure if any two of the methods were correlated.

Table 4. Linear Regression Summary of Figures 1, 2, and 3 with Temperature and Relative Humidity Parameters

	Univariate Slope (SD)	Univariate Model R^2	Multivariate[‡] Slope (SE)	Multivariate[‡] Model R^2
NIOSH vs RKI[*]				
Intercept (model w/RKI)	0.098 (0.032)		−2.643 (1.067)	
RKI	0.957 (0.076)	0.780	0.884 (0.080)	
Temperature	−0.031 (0.007)	0.280	−0.017 (0.008)	
Relative Humidity	0.028 (0.005)	0.348	0.019 (0.006)	
Error Variance			0.022	0.829
NIOSH vs PPM[*]				
Intercept (model w/ PPM)	0.0959 (0.028)		0.643 (0.266)	
PPM	1.368 (0.067)	0.902	1.282 (0.069)	
Temperature[†]	−0.031 (0.007)	0.280	−0.008 (0.003)	
	—	—	—	
Error Variance			0.010	0.917

[*]NIOSH as dependent variable, RKI and PPM as independent variables
[†]Relative humidity omitted, as not significant, minor improvement in R^2 (0.919)
[‡]In all multivariate models, temperature and relative humidity showed evidence of collinearity with the intercept.

For the purpose of this study, sensitivity and specificity were defined with an arbitrary value. The observations were concentrated at and below 0.2 ppm on the scatter plots; therefore, 0.2 ppm was picked as the arbitrary value for the sensitivity and specificity calculations. The sensitivity is the probability of a true positive value above 0.2 ppm, whereas the specificity is the probability of a false positive value below 0.2 ppm. For detecting a formaldehyde level above 0.2 ppm according to NIOSH Method 2016, the RKI Instruments Model FP-30 had 60% sensitivity and 92% specificity. The receiver operating characteristic (ROC) curve is a plot of the true positive values against the false positive values. The area under the ROC curve based on logistic regression was 0.886 for the RKI Instruments Model FP-30. For the PPM Technology Formaldemeter™ *htV* to detect a formaldehyde level above 0.2 ppm, the sensitivity was 88% and the specificity was 65%. The area under the ROC curve based on logistic regression was 0.910 for the PPM Technology Formaldemeter™ *htV*.

Temperature and Relative Humidity

Temperatures in the THUs ranged from 80°F–102°F with an average temperature of 89°F. Relative humidity ranged from 50%–83% with an average reading of 67%. Relative humidity was positively associated with formaldehyde concentrations for all three methods, whereas ambient temperature was negatively associated with the methods.

DISCUSSION

The purpose of this study was to compare two commercially available direct-reading instruments with NIOSH Method 2016. The means of the integrated formaldehyde measurements obtained using the direct-reading instruments were positively correlated with measurements obtained using NIOSH Method 2016 ($R^2 = 0.780$ for RKI Instruments Model FP-30 and 0.902 for PPM Technology Formaldemeter™ *htV*). However, the RKI Instruments Model FP-30 method ($p < 0.001$) yielded statistically significantly lower readings than NIOSH Method 2016, whereas the differences, on average with the PPM Technology Formaldemeter™ *htV* ($p = 0.15$) were not statistically significantly different from NIOSH Method 2016.

All three scatter plots showed a positive correlation between the different types of formaldehyde measurements. Both direct-reading instruments had a higher positive correlation with the NIOSH Method ($R^2 = 0.780$ for RKI Instruments Model FP-30 and 0.902 for PPM Technology

Formaldemeter™ *htV*) than with each other ($R^2 = 0.699$). The Bland-Altman plots suggested little pattern in the differences between the three methods other than possibly greater variation at higher values.

Approximately 78% of the variability in the RKI Instruments Model FP-30 results is accounted for by a linear relationship with NIOSH Method 2016 sample collection results (Table 2). According to the manufacturer, the high temperature and relative humidity readings from this study should not have caused a background reading on the instrument [RKI Instruments 2003]. Of the variability in the PPM Technology Formaldemeter™ *htV* results, 90% is accounted for by a linear relationship with NIOSH Method 2016 data (Table 2). The PPM Technology Formaldemeter™ *htV* was calibrated each day in the morning when temperatures and relative humidity were within the recommended parameters. Because both temperature (89°F) and relative humidity (67%) were above the favorable operating range, the reliability of the PPM instrument's formaldehyde readings was a concern with higher formaldehyde readings than reported by the monitor.

For this study, temperature was no longer significant, after accounting for relative humidity's correlation to NIOSH Method 2016. There was a negative association of NIOSH Method 2016 with temperature (e.g., as temperature increased, NIOSH Method 2016 formaldehyde readings decreased). This negative association could have been caused by the ventilated condition as the temperature inside the THUs increased. As the temperature in the THUs increased, the doors and windows of the THUs were opened. This change in ventilation state may have confounded

23

with the temperatures in the THUs causing the temperature to have no importance as a parameter in data analysis.

Sensitivity and specificity tests showed that the PPM Technology Formaldemeter™ *htV* was better at predicting formaldehyde concentrations greater than 0.2 ppm compared to the RKI Instruments Model FP-30. Temperature and ventilation state may have affected each instrument's ability to detect formaldehyde levels greater than the arbitrary value of 0.2 ppm.

According to the manufacturer, the PPM Technology Formaldemeter™ *htV* monitor requires regular calibration to guarantee the monitor is functioning properly. The formaldehyde calibration standard, thermometer, and temperature/concentration table are used to check and adjust the calibration of the instrument. However, the thermometer supplied with the PPM Technology Formaldemeter™ *htV* monitor is difficult to use and could affect the accuracy of the monitor's calibration. Accurate readings from the thermometer are needed because formaldehyde concentrations in the calibration standard vary with temperature [PPM Technology Ltd 2005]. Additionally, the temperature/concentration table is only useful for temperatures in the range of 59°F–84°F. Because the highest temperatures in this field study were outside the recommended range, the readings from the PPM Technology Formaldemeter™ *htV* monitor may not have been accurate. This temperature difference was a weakness for this field study because, according to the temperature/concentration table, a one degree change in temperature means more than a 10% difference in concentration.

One potential drawback of the RKI Instruments Model FP-30 monitor is its inability to report formaldehyde concentrations greater than 1.00 ppm. In some applications this could be a major issue, but for screening to detect elevated levels (e.g., greater than 0.2 ppm), this should pose little or no problem. The monitor gives a reading of "over," if the concentration measured is greater than 1.00 ppm. The five RKI Instruments Model FP-30 readings that were above the monitor's limit would have been greater than 1.00 ppm if a value had been reported.

Other weaknesses of this field study included the lack of precision (the instruments may have varied independently of the variation in the NIOSH reference method). A reference method is a benchmark and research standards preclude the altering of the benchmark, which was another weakness in the study. Therefore, the NIOSH Method 2016 could not be manipulated in this study. Not being able to use 25 of the 72 sample results in the analysis was another weakness since it decreased the sample size and therefore the ability to detect statistical differences. Pump calibration issues and the operation of PPM Technology Formaldemeter™ htV instrument above its recommended temperature range were other weaknesses in this study. Despite the weaknesses, the field study provided a realistic test environment and flexibility to compare the different methods.

CONCLUSIONS

The 1-hour integrated sample collected with the RKI Instruments Model FP-30 was statistically significantly different from the NIOSH Method 2016 ($p<0.001$), whereas the 1-hour integrated sample collected with the PPM Technology Formaldemeter™ htV was not statistically significantly different from the NIOSH Method ($p=0.15$). High temperature and relative humidity readings, the direct-reading instruments' operating capability and environment sensitivity, and pump pre- and post-sampling flow rate differences greater than 10% may have affected the relationship between the instruments and NIOSH Method 2016. Under the test situations, the PPM Technology Formaldemeter™ *htV* had similar, though slightly better, discriminatory ability for detecting formaldehyde concentrations over 0.2 ppm compared to the RKI Instruments Model FP-30, based on the area under the ROC curve and a 1-hour integrated sample.

Although the direct-reading instruments differed from NIOSH Method 2016, scatter plots and correlation tests showed that the 1-hour integrated sample collected with the instruments correlated with those from the laboratory-based method. A 1-hour integrated sample collected with the direct-reading instruments maybe useful as screening tools and might preclude the need for timely and expensive laboratory analysis if low concentrations are measured. However, additional field evaluations under a variety of environmental conditions and formaldehyde concentrations are needed to better understand the accuracy of these direct-reading instruments as compared to NIOSH Method 2016.

REFERENCES

ATSDR [1999]. Agency for Toxic Substances and Disease Registry toxicological profile for formaldehyde. Atlanta, GA: U.S. Department of Health and Human Services, Centers for Disease Control and Prevention, Agency for Toxic Substances and Disease Registry. [www.atsdr.cdc.gov/toxprofiles/tp111.html]. Date accessed: May 2009.

Hornung RW, Reed LD [1990]. Estimation of average concentration in the presence of nondetectable values. Appl Occup Environ Hyg *5*(1):46–51.

Kelly TJ, Smith DL, Satola J [1999]. Emission rates of formaldehyde from materials and consumer products found in California homes. Environ Sci Tech *33*(1):81–88.

Khoder MI, Shakour AA, Farag SA, Abdel Hameed AA [2000]. Indoor and outdoor formaldehyde concentrations in homes in residential areas in Greater Cairo. J Environ Monit *2*(2):123–126.

NIOSH [1995]. Guidelines for air sampling and analytical method development and evaluation. Washington, DC: U.S. Department of Health and Human Services, Centers for Disease Control and Prevention, National Institute for Occupational Safety and Health, DHHS (NIOSH) Publication No. 95-117. [www.cdc.gov/niosh/docs/95-117/]. Date accessed: May 2009.

NIOSH [2003]. Formaldehyde: Method 2016 (supplement issued 01/15/1998). In: Eller PM, Cassinelli ME, eds. NIOSH manual of analytical methods. 4th ed. Cincinnati, OH: U.S. Department of Health and Human Services, Centers for Disease Control and Prevention, National Institute for Occupational Safety and Health, DHHS (NIOSH) Publication No. 94-113. [www.cdc.gov/niosh/nmam/]. Date accessed: May 2009.

NIOSH [2005]. Pocket guide to chemical hazards. Cincinnati, OH: U.S. Department of Health and Human Services, Centers for Disease Control and Prevention, National Institute for Occupational Safety and Health, DHHS (NIOSH) Publication No. 2005-149. [www.cdc.gov/niosh/npg/]. Date accessed: May 2009.

Peluffo S (speluffo@rkiinstruments.com) [2009]. RKI Tech Support Web Inquiry. Private e-mail message to RKI Instruments, Inc. (support@rkiinstruments.com), April 22.

Pickrell JA, Mokier BV, Griffis LC, Hobbs CH [1983]. Formaldehyde release rate coefficients from selected consumer products. Environ Sci Tech *17*(12):753–757.

PPM Technology Ltd [2005]. PPM Formaldemeter™ *htV* 3 parameter IAQ monitor operation manual. Caernarfon: Wales, UK.

RKI Instruments Inc [2003]. Instruction manual for formaldehyde gas detector model FP-30/FP-40. Hayward, CA.

Roberts L (laura@ppm-technology.com) [2009]. Formaldemeter questions. Private e-mail message to PPM Technology Ltd (technical@ppm-technology.com), April 22.

Sexton K, Petreas MX, Liu K [1989]. Formaldehyde exposures inside mobile homes. Am Chem Soc *23*(8):985–988.

U.S. Consumer Product Safety Commission [1997]. An update on formaldehyde-1997 revision. [www.cpsc.gov/cpscpub/pubs/725.html]. Date accessed: May 2009.

APPENDIX

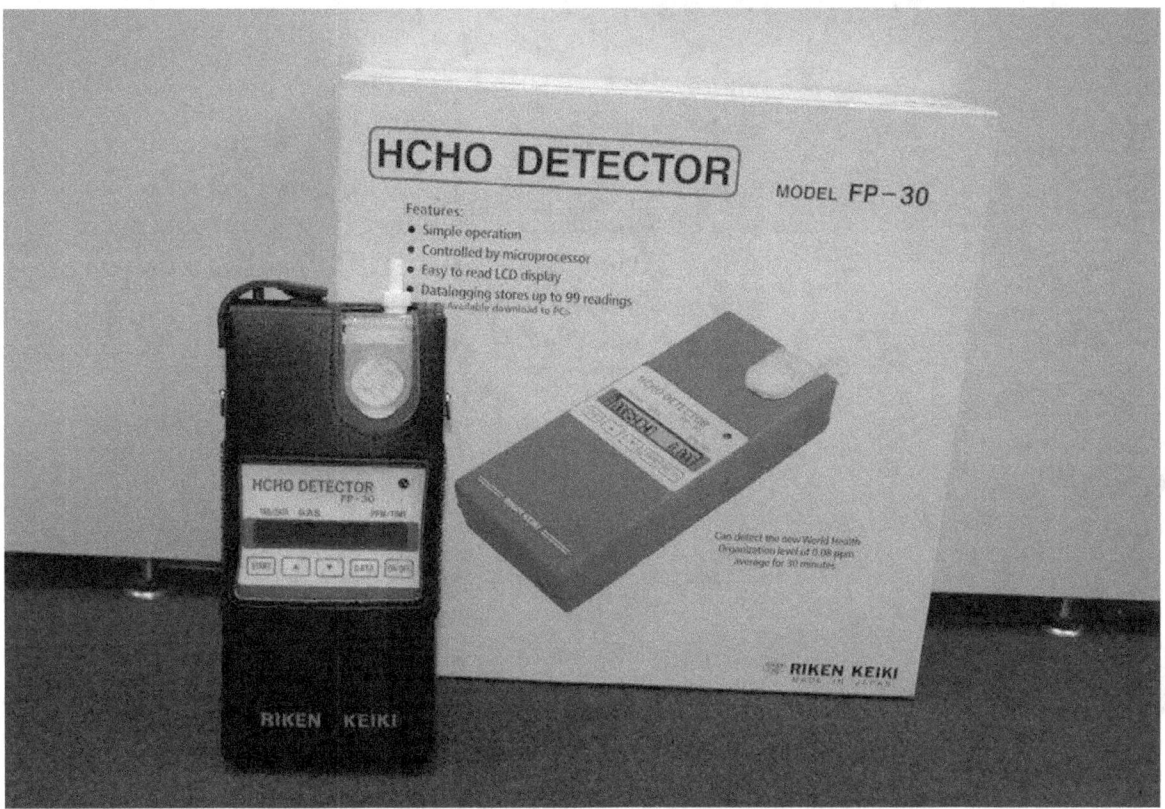

Figure A-1. RKI Instruments Model FP-30

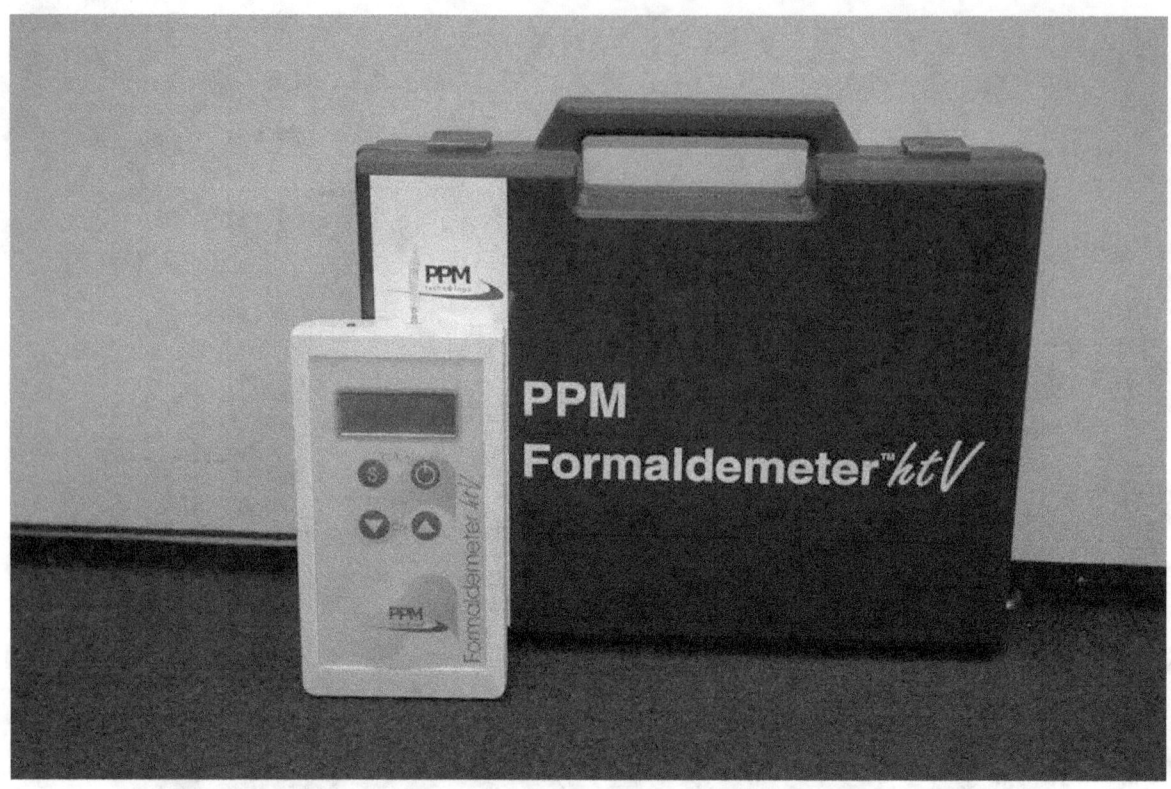

Figure A-2. PPM Technology Formaldemeter™ *htV*

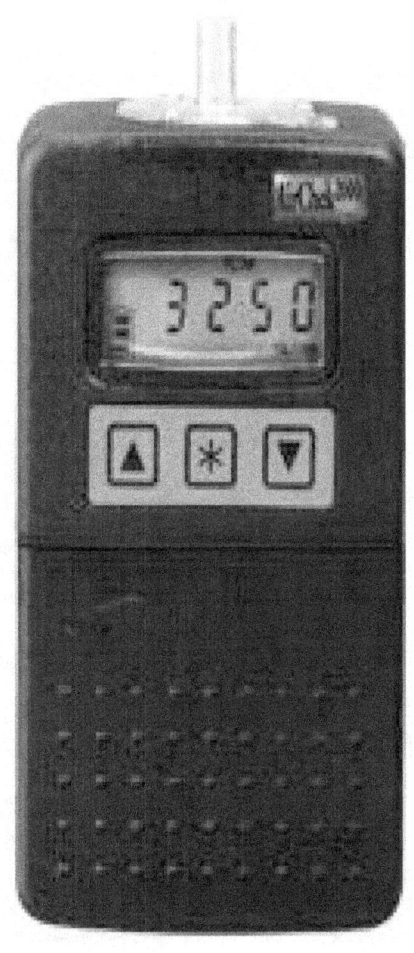

Figure A-3. SKC AirCheck® 2000

Figure A–4. Sample Data Sheet Page 1

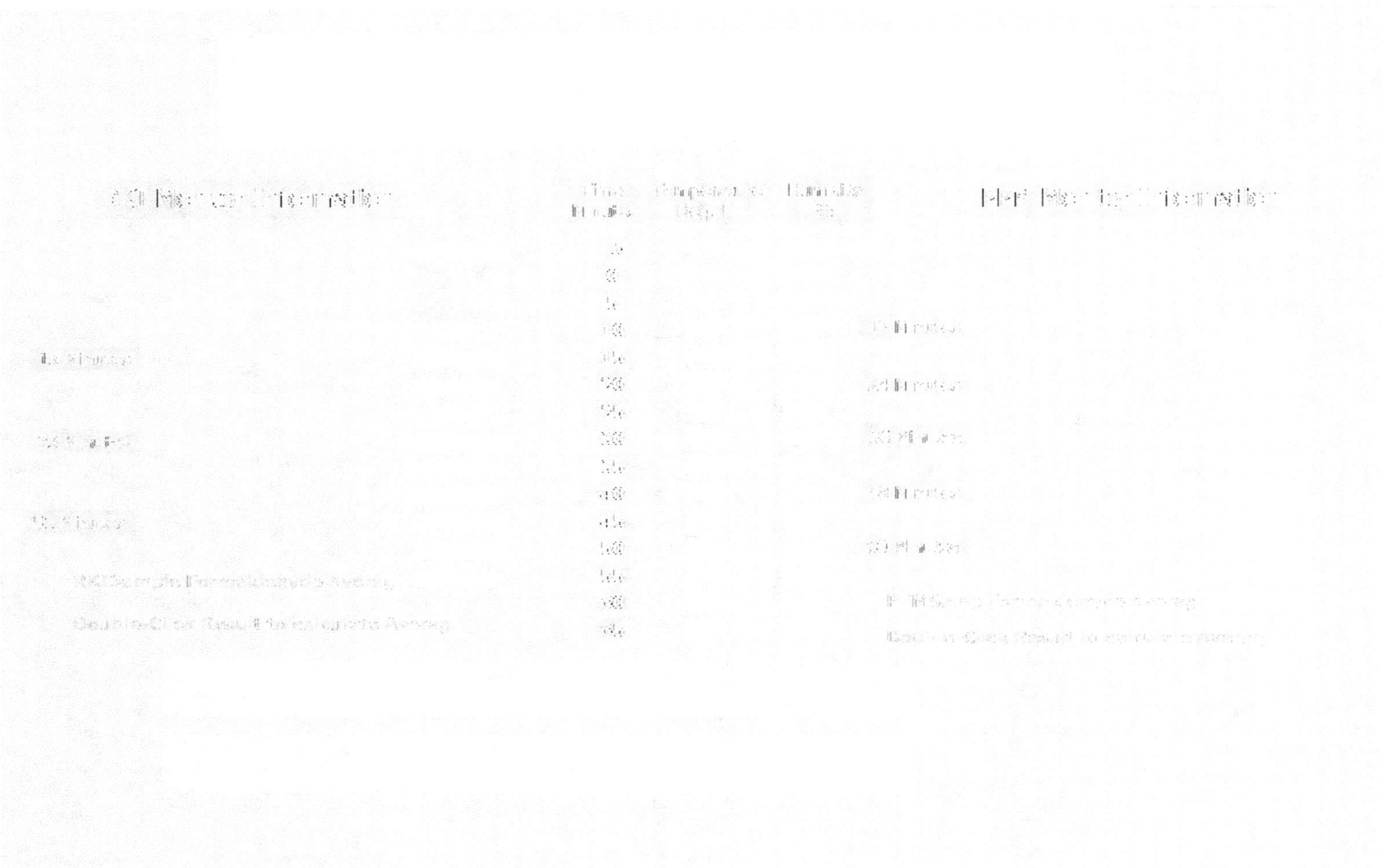

Figure A-5. Sample Data Sheet Page 2

33

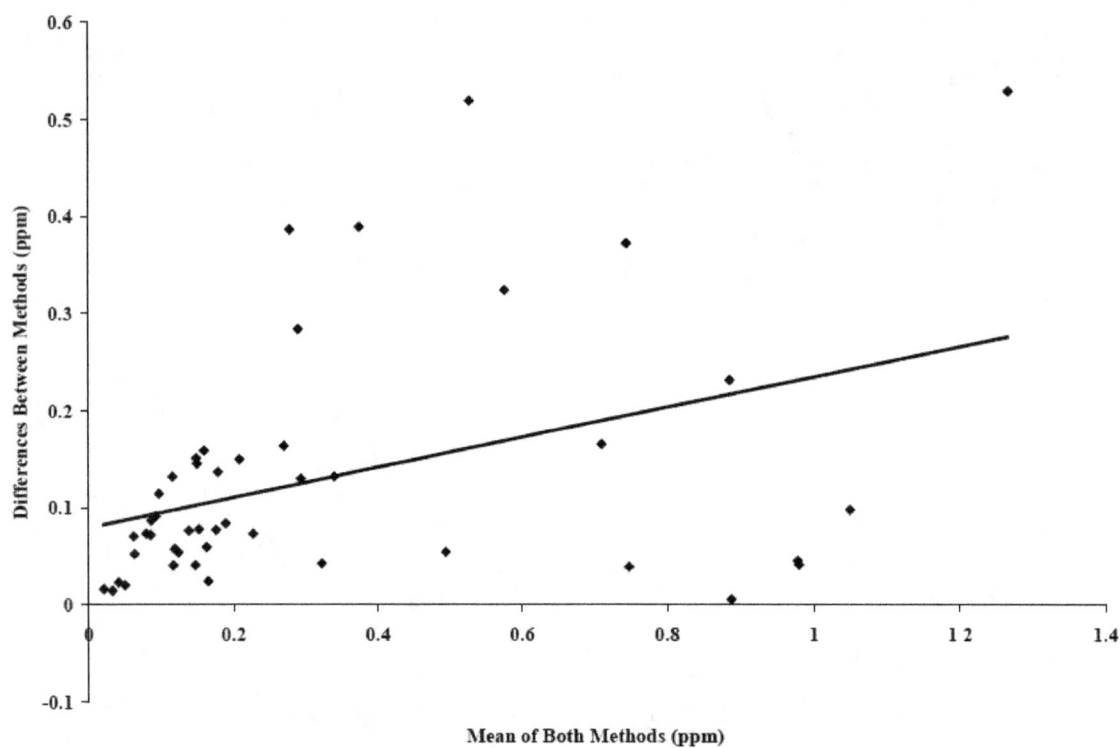

Figure A-6. Mean of NIOSH Method 2016 and RKI Instruments Model FP-30. Bland-Altman plot of the data obtained from 47 paired samples measured with NIOSH Method 2016 and RKI Instruments Model FP-30. Correlation R = 0.3898 (p<0.01). Slope = 0.1553 (p<0.01). Intercept = 0.0795 (p<0.01).

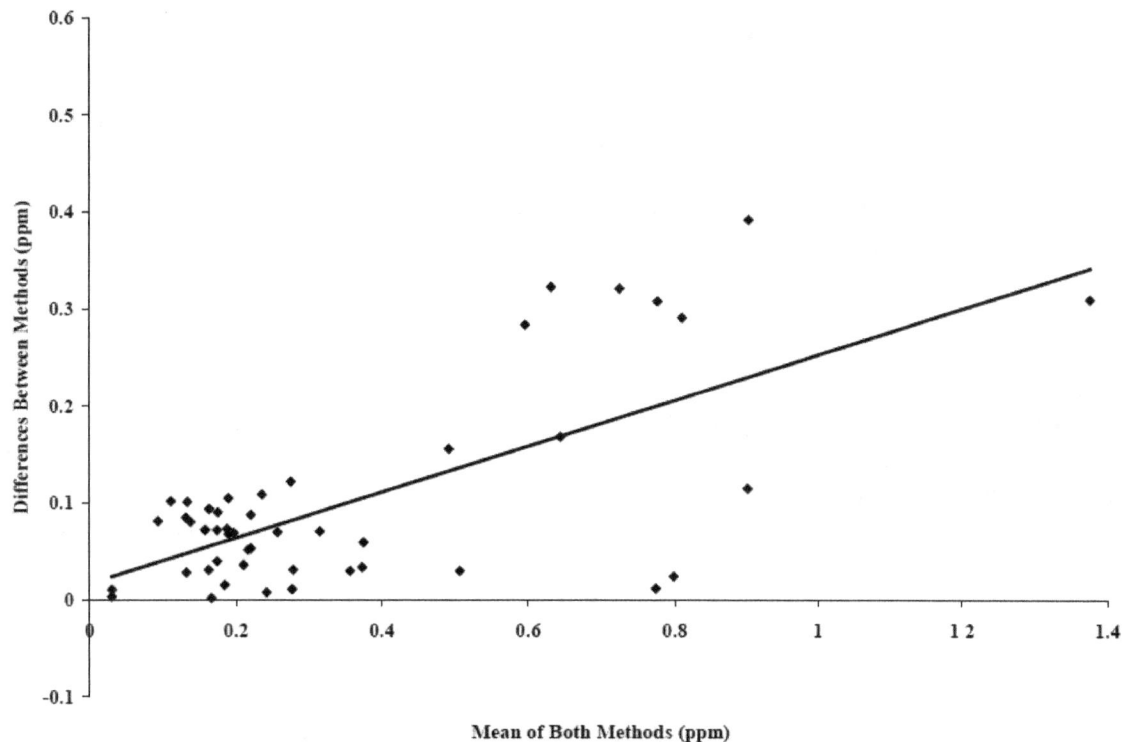

Figure A-7. Mean of NIOSH Method 2016 and PPM Technology Formaldemeter™ *htV*. Bland-Altman plot of the data obtained from 47 paired samples measured with NIOSH Method 2016 and PPM Technology Formaldemeter™ *htV*. Correlation R = 0.6798 (p<0.01). Slope = 0.2363 (p<0.01). Intercept = 0.0163 (p=0.35).

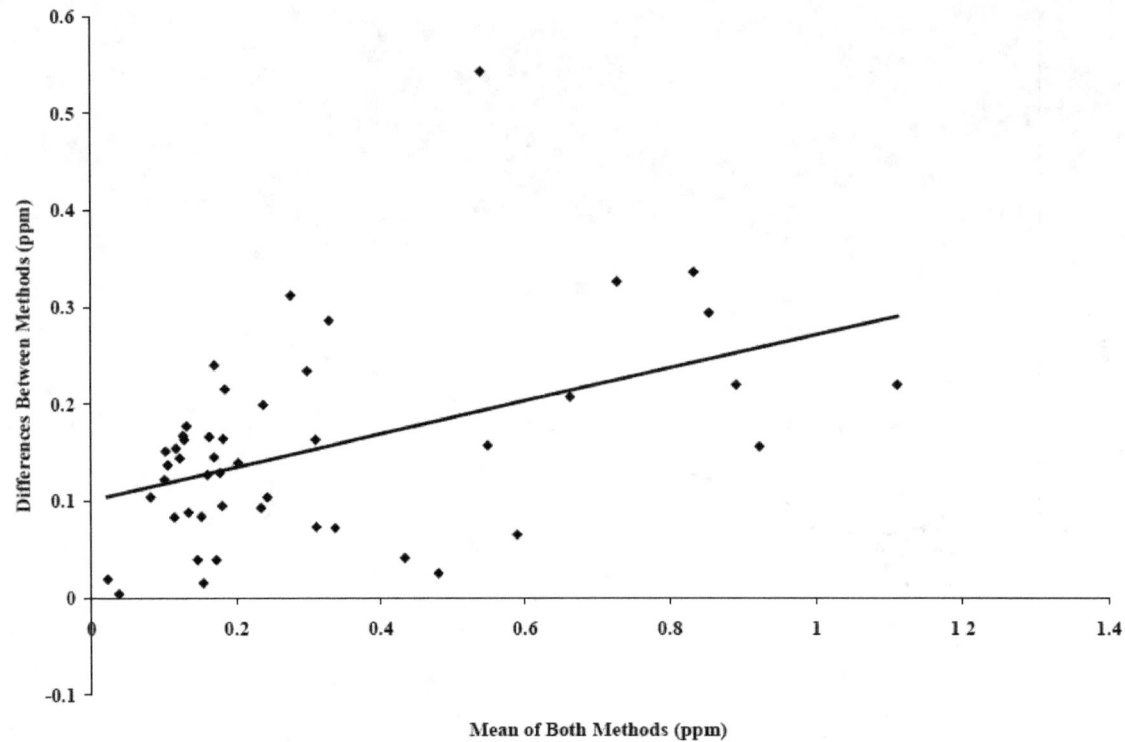

Figure A-8. Mean RKI Instruments Model FP-30 and PPM Technology Formaldemeter™ *htV*. Bland-Altman plot of the data obtained from 47 paired samples measured with RKI Instruments Model FP-30 and PPM Technology Formaldemeter™ *htV*. Correlation R = 0.4508 (p<0.01). Slope = 0.1710 (p<0.01). Intercept = 0.1005 (p<0.01).

Table A-1. Summary Statistics for NIOSH, RKI, and PPM Sampling Methods

Method Paired Triplets	N	Mean (SD) (ppm)	Mean Difference vs NIOSH (SD) (ppm)	Min / Max (ppm)
NIOSH	72	0.37 (0.34)	—	0.0014 / 1.5
RKI	72	0.26 (0.29)	0.11 (0.050)	0.013 / 1.00
PPM	72	0.349 (0.250)	0.0210 (0.0900)	0.0320 / 1.270

Table A- 2. Summary Statistics for NIOSH, RKI, and PPM Sampling Methods for Sample Results Greater than 1

Method Paired Triplets	N	Mean (SD) (ppm)	Mean Difference vs NIOSH (SD) (ppm)	Min / Max (ppm)
NIOSH	5	1.1 (0.29)	—	0.77 / 1.5
RKI	5	1.00 (0.00)	0.10 (0.29)	1.00 / 1.00
PPM	5	0.843 (0.222)	0.257 (0.068)	0.664 / 1.220